MW01260070

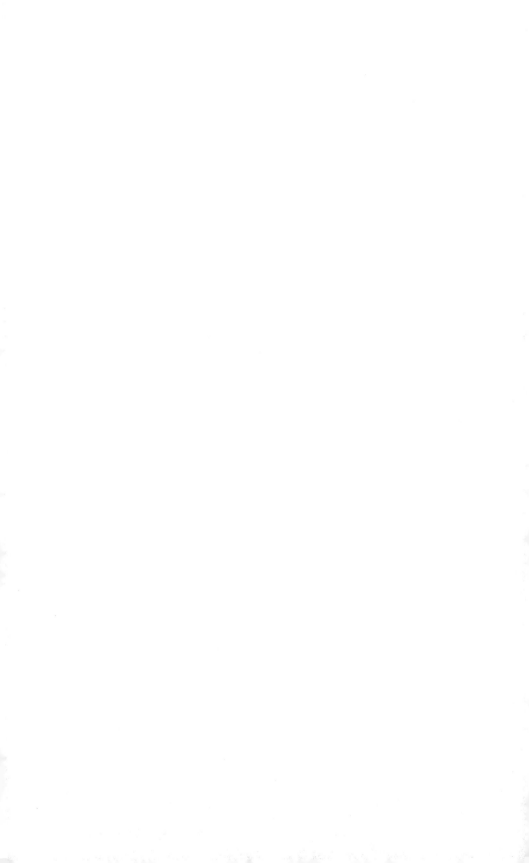

# Better Health

## And a Plan to Achieve It

The Dawning of a New Day and a New You

Hugh H. Bassham

WESTBOW
PRESS®
A DIVISION OF THOMAS NELSON
& ZONDERVAN

Scripture taken from the HOLY BIBLE, NEW INTERNATIONAL VERSION®. Copyright © 1973, 1978, 1984 Biblica. Used by permission of Zondervan. All rights reserved.

WestBow Press books may be ordered through booksellers or by contacting:

WestBow Press
A Division of Thomas Nelson & Zondervan
1663 Liberty Drive
Bloomington, IN 47403
www.westbowpress.com
1 (866) 928-1240

ISBN: 978-1-4908-9841-4 (sc)
ISBN: 978-1-4908-9842-1 (e)

Library of Congress Control Number: 2015917484

Print information available on the last page.

WestBow Press rev. date: 10/15/2015

To my grandson,
Matthew

# Contents

# Introduction

As a veterinarian, I have learned much from the animals I worked with. And the more I learned from them, the more I realized I could apply this knowledge to people. Eventually, as I felt more and more accountable for what I had learned, I wrote a book, *The Search for Total Health,* which was published in 1993.

Knowledge and understanding is one thing, but *applying* that knowledge and understanding is another. So in 2007 I wrote a booklet, *A Plan for Better Health,* hoping it would help, not only with understanding, but with applying this understanding in a practical and useful way.

Now, in 2010, I have combined these two works, the book and the booklet, under a new title, *Better Health and a Plan to Achieve It.* It is my hope that this book will help us all understand, and achieve, better health.

*Hugh H. Bassham*
Quitman, Georgia
September 24, 2009

# Acknowledgement:

This book is a reality because of the counsel and support of many friends. I thank you all.

I would also like to thank CrossBooks Publishing and the CrossBooks Team for all they have done, and for going the extra mile.

**Part One**

———

# The Search For Total Health

# Foreword

**M**odern man is searching for many things: financial security, comfort, happiness, freedom from anxiety, world peace, and even good health. But is he searching for total health? Is he even interested in it? Does he even know what constitutes total health?

How is it that a well-conditioned athlete at the zenith of his physical capabilities takes a gun and kills himself? Most would say that he was in excellent health, but I would say that he had not achieved total health. How is it that a prayerful, deeply committed minister of the gospel suddenly drops dead from a heart attack at age forty? Most would say that his spiritual health was superb, but I would say that he had not achieved total health.

The athlete thought he could condition his body while ignoring the condition of his soul. The minister thought that he could care for his soul while ignoring his physical conditioning. Both were wrong. Both fell short of the ultimate abundance of life that was available to them. Both should have been concerned about their outward *and* inward conditions. Both should have been searching for a state of total health.

The search for total health begins with a humble heart and an open mind. But this is not always easy, especially when it comes to accepting and acting upon ideas that are new and perhaps controversial. But let us remember that over the course of history, new and different ideas have rarely been embraced quickly by the masses. Nevertheless, to progress as individuals and as a society, we must be willing to consider new and different ideas, remembering that all ideas were at one time new and different.

To get the most out of this book, it must be read with a thoughtful and inquiring mind. It is the author's intention to not only present some interesting and useful ideas, but also to inspire the reader to an attitude of pondering and questioning, thereby provoking a search for much more than this modest book proposes to communicate.

This book is only intended as a beginning. Its purpose is to provide a foundation upon which a person can build with confidence. The Bible says that a wise man builds on a solid foundation. I have done my utmost to construct this foundation to be solid.

By being short, this book can easily be read and reread. It can be pondered until the principles it presents become ingrained in the reader's mind. Through thoughtful, even prayerful consideration, I believe understanding can be acquired. This understanding, when followed by determined, decisive action, will help us reach the goal that I believe we should all be searching for: total health.

## Chapter 1

# Total Human Health

Of the many needs facing our society, the need for good health is one of the most important. The poorer the health of a nation, the poorer the nation. If we want a prosperous society, the search for the keys to sound, enduring health ought to be a top priority. Instead, it has been my observation that many people take the state of their health for granted and become concerned about it only when it begins to deteriorate. Wouldn't it be better if we practiced those things that promote good health rather than struggling to restore it once it is lost? I see the promoting and maintaining of good health to be the "wave of the future." This wave can already be seen in the increasing interest in our society in proper diet and exercise. With medical costs rising and diseases such as cancer and heart disease constantly increasing, many people have become concerned about preserving their good health for as long as possible.

Though many individuals are beginning to take steps to improve their own personal health, beyond that, I believe we need to see a drastic change in direction in our society as a whole. I would like to see our emphasis change from one of diagnosing and treating disease to one of preventing it altogether. I recognize that there will always be a need for some level of diagnosis and treatment. To propose that we could ever eliminate it altogether would be excessive idealism. But why couldn't the main thrust of our efforts be redirected toward prevention of disease, or to put it better, preservation of good health?

For a long time now we have suffered from what I call the Ten-Ninety Syndrome (TNS): we have put ten percent of our effort into preserving health and ninety percent into treating disease. In other words, we have given most of our attention to something we don't want—disease— and very little attention to something we do want—good health. The assumption has been that by studying and understanding disease, we will be better able to understand and achieve good health. This concept is only partially valid. I agree that we must know something about our enemy if we are to defeat it, but it is possible to concentrate so excessively on the enemy that he actually becomes stronger through our own neglect of the things that maintain our strength. As long as we do this, victory will continually elude us.

Fortunately, there is a simple solution to the problem of TNS: simply reverse the percentages! Why not spend ninety percent of our time looking for ways to encourage and preserve good health and only ten percent on diagnosing and treating disease? Admittedly this is somewhat of an over-simplification; but what I am really proposing is that we need a change of attitude. We should be emphasizing what we want rather than what we don't want.

## The Foundation

So where do we begin? Well, when a contractor gets ready to erect a building, he begins by constructing a solid foundation. To construct a lifetime of good health, we must begin by considering what constitutes the foundation of good health. According to the Greek physician Hippocrates, who is known as the Father of Medicine, "Nutrition is the foundation of health." Hippocrates made this statement nearly 2,500 years ago, and it has stood the test of time. Yet even Hippocrates was not the first to recognize the relationship between the quality of the food we eat and good health, for nearly one thousand years before Hippocrates, Moses wrote, "Worship the Lord your God, and His blessing will be on your food and water. I will take away sickness from among you" (Exodus 23:25).

Therefore, to announce that there is a relationship between proper nutrition and good health is nothing new. Neither is it new or controversial to say that malnutrition leads to poor health, or that the better the quality of the nourishment, the better the health. These facts have been known and accepted for generations. But I believe that it's time for us as a society to begin in earnest to concentrate on promoting good nutrition. Could it be that much of the disease in the world is present solely because people are not nourishing themselves as they should?

Let's take a closer look at nutrition and attempt to discover just how profoundly it really does impact our health. And not only ours as human beings, but also the health of animals and plants, since we are partners in God's complex ecological system. And let us also consider that there just may be more to the issue of nutrition than that which comes to us from the earth. Jesus Christ said that man does not live on bread alone, "but on every word that comes from the mouth of God" (Matthew 4:4). There is a spiritual nutrition that comes from God for our souls.

Some have believed that they only needed to be concerned with providing proper nutrition to their physical man, but Jesus has informed us that if we are to truly live, we must also provide proper nutrition to our spiritual man. Some have tried to live by bread alone. Other well-meaning people have thought that they could live by God's Word alone. The truth is, to achieve total health, that is, the maximum wholeness and fitness of the total person that God has made available for each individual, we must be concerned about both.

Before we go on, allow me to make one further comment. I have written this book from a Christian perspective. When I speak of good and evil, right and wrong, strong and weak, I speak using the Bible as my standard of measurement. That which is good is not good according to my opinion, but good according to biblical values and principles.

To those Christians who are reading this book and wondering if my thesis has any special application to those of the household of faith, my answer is most assuredly, yes! Christ is our Healer to be sure; but even greater than His ability to heal us is His ability to preserve us and sustain us. I believe that He receives far greater glory in the preservation of the health of His people than He does in their being healed. Unfortunately, many believers have been unaware of some basic principles concerning the preservation of good health and have fallen into the pit of physical weakness and disease.

Certainly the Lord was lamenting when He said, "My people are destroyed from lack of knowledge" (Hosea 4:6). To expect the Lord to sustain our health, we must have knowledge of His foundational principles of health. As knowledge increases, however, often perplexity increases right along with it. How can anyone possibly keep up with every new discovery, every new idea brought to light?

## Specialization vs. Generalization

Some suggest that the answer lies in specialization. But my observation has been that over the course of time, specializations tend to focus primarily on the part, the specialty, while neglecting the whole, which is the underlying reason for the specialization in the first place. I am not opposed to specialization per se; only suggesting that we be careful that as we strive to progress, we don't lose sight of our ultimate goal. Perhaps it is generalization, not specialization, that really needs the greater emphasis. Allow me to explain why I feel this way.

The human body is composed of many distinct yet interdependent parts; the heart, the lungs, the liver, the kidneys, and so forth. To consider one part without considering its relationship to the body as a whole is to run the risk of compounding the problem. Yet this happens frequently. The treatment of one health problem ends up bringing on another problem, if not immediately, then down the road. Specialization is only valid when practiced in light of the whole.

To take this concept one step further, to treat the physical body without consideration of the spiritual dimension is to risk doing more harm than good. Jesus said, "You foolish people! Did not the one who made the outside make the inside also?" (Luke 11:40). Yet when the word "health" is mentioned, inevitably most people (especially those in the medical community) think immediately of the physical body. But no human being can function in a state of total health over the long-term unless consideration is given to both the outward and the inward man. There are specific nutritional requirements for the outward man, and there are equally specific nutritional requirements for the inward man. Specializations in just one or the other won't do.

If we as a society have any hope of providing a more successful approach to achieving total and lasting health, we must establish a better nutritional foundation. Knowledge may increase and specialization may be modified and perfected, but a truly solid foundation should be characterized by stability and permanence; it should not be subject to periodic adjustments and improvements. The problem for many of us is that foundations are not very exciting. They are, however, vitally important. Nothing intended to last a lifetime should be erected upon a weak or shaky foundation. For this reason, let us look at the basic nutritional requirements of both the outward and the inward parts of man. My hope and prayer is that this book will carry us all forward toward a more accurate understanding and, of course, better health.

## Chapter 2

# The Nourishment of the Outward Man

I am convinced that most people know intuitively that physical health necessitates a proper and balanced diet. The problem is, the modern lifestyles of man are not conducive to good eating habits. Even when we make a well-intentioned effort to eat correctly, many of us still continue to suffer debilitating illnesses due essentially to malnutrition. Thus, a nutrition-poor, toxin-infested diet, whether consumed knowingly or unknowingly, is the most blatant cause of chronic poor health in our society and the world at large today.

The global victims of extreme emaciation are the more conspicuous results of gross malnutrition. Well-documented deficiency diseases such as beriberi, pellagra, and rickets continue to claim thousands of lives in the Third World. Most have heard of the classic case of the sailors plagued with scurvy. This disease was suddenly and completely cured upon the discovery that it was caused by an ascorbic acid (vitamin C) deficiency. The simple addition of lemon juice to the sailor's diet eliminated the plague. Many have seen the pictures of rats on vitamin-deficient diets and how they compare to rats on a normal diet. Or the pictures of chickens on a mineral-deficient diet and the dramatic comparison with chickens on a normal diet. Such graphic illustrations of the effects of poor nutrition can be found in most encyclopedias. They vividly demonstrate the severe damage that can be inflicted by a simple vitamin or mineral deficiency.

Many of us might smile and think to ourselves that this was all a long time ago and that things are different now. But are they? My belief is that we are laboring under a false sense of security. Malnutrition in various forms and its resultant deficiency diseases are still very much with us, and probably to a greater degree then ever before. How can this be the case when we have supposedly made such progress in fighting disease?

I believe that if we could accurately trace every disease to its roots, we would discover that there is really only one disease: malnutrition. All other diseases are simply symptom complexes springing from this lone root. Could this really be true? To some of you this may seem far-fetched, even naive. But in spite of what some traditionalists may claim, I am convinced that all disease is in some way connected to malnutrition.

## The Food We Eat

Have you ever read a pet food container that said, "100% nutritionally complete"? Or have you ever been told that good health depends on eating a "balanced diet"? Is it really that simple? Is it possible for any pet food to be 100% nutritionally complete for the average dog in the average situation, whatever that may be? And what really constitutes a "balanced diet" for a human being? Does anyone really know for sure? It is interesting and not uncommon for the United States government to revise what it considers to be a balanced diet. How comprehensive, then, is our understanding of the nutritional needs of humans and animals? As a veterinarian, I can testify that our understanding is extremely limited.

If good nutrition were as easily obtained as some advertising campaigns would have us believe, then where is all this disease coming from? Some would answer that it's coming from germs—microorganisms such as bacteria or viruses. But I submit to you that germs are only a secondary cause. Haven't you ever wondered why a "bug" can be going around and some people catch it while others don't? What is it that determines the strength or weakness of a person's immune system? To a large extent, it is nutrition. I believe that the closer a person approaches what I call total health, the less power germs have to produce disease and influence strength or weakness. Germs come up against an impenetrable wall when a person's outward and inward man are receiving proper nourishment.

The "100% complete" label implies absolute perfection and total knowledge. But has science really advanced to the point where we can say with confidence that everything is known about physiology, digestion or biochemistry? Actually, the case is quite the contrary. Nutrition is probably our most inexact science. For decades, the study of nutrition has lagged behind other fields of study. But this has not been because of its simplicity or its lack of importance. Actually, it has probably been because of its complexity, for to fully understand the science of nutrition one must have a detailed understanding of nearly every other branch of science. This, needless to say, is a monumental task which few have endeavored to master.

Often it is the effect of very subtle imbalances, excesses or deficiencies that make the difference in health, especially long-term health. Just because a food doesn't cause immediate and obvious harm in the short term does not mean it will be beneficial over the long term. In fact, seemingly minor changes in health that occur at a young age often never become clinically recognizable until a much older age. Disease does not always descend upon us suddenly as it sometimes seems. More often it is the result of a long-term process involving many factors and shortfalls. The outward manifestation as a symptom complex is the only thing sudden about most diseases.

This brings us to some crucial questions: If proper nutrition is so vital yet so complicated, and if nutritional science is still only just emerging, what are we to do to maximize the state of our health? What are we to eat? When we go to the supermarket, how are we to know which foods are good for us and which should be avoided?

## Natural Foods

Fortunately, these difficult questions have a simple answer: as much as possible, we should eat natural foods. By natural I mean foods which are grown, harvested, and prepared without excessive human intervention. Foods left under the dominion of nature have sustained life on this planet since the beginning of time. It has only been in recent times that modern food technology has confused us into believing that man can improve upon what God has created. But I ask, is this really within the scope of man's capabilities? Advertisements may extol the virtues of the "vitamin enriched, low fat, low cholesterol" foods we see in our stores, but are they as good for us as those served up without extensive processing? We must be wary of such claims.

A simple potato, for example, contains over one hundred fifty chemically distinct entities, and does anyone really know how each of these or any combination of these is significant in the maximizing of our health? Doesn't it make sense to simply trust that the Lord knows all the details of our bodies' nutritional needs? We don't have to figure it all out; we simply need to eat what the Lord has provided. An apple, a carrot and a filet mignon each contain trace elements in various configurations which may never be fully understood or appreciated by man. How can we ever be sure that man's "improvements" are really a benefit to our health? It seems to me that for man, with his new knowledge and new technology, to claim superiority over God and nature is arrogant indeed. Besides, that portion of man's technology which is valid and truly useful is nothing more than the discovery of laws and principles established by God in the first place. It is at best only a crude representation of the infinite knowledge of God. Thus, it is God who is the ultimate source of knowledge and designer of technology.

The superiority of the natural, archetypal diet over the modern, purified, fractionated, processed diet has been demonstrated over and over again. Studies by Dr. Francis Pottenger in the 1930s showed the superiority of non-heated foods over their heated counterparts. Anthropological studies have demonstrated that the diets of many primitive peoples, when duplicated today, will tend to produce a general state of good health. The health of a society tends to deteriorate, however, when modern processed foods such as white sugar, white flour, white salt and white oils (which I consider to be the four white poisons) become dietary staples.

Over the past few years, large statistical studies have suggested a clear link between the consumption of processed foods and a variety of degenerative diseases, including cancer, heart disease, allergies, arthritis, obesity and dental disease. Therefore, the admonition now is to increase the intake of fiber, fresh fruits, fresh vegetables and lean meats, which we have every reason to believe will decrease the incidence of these and other diseases in our society. In other words, in our battle against disease, good nutrition, in the form of natural foods, should be the point of the spear.

## The Original Diet

Our goal as individuals and as a society should be to duplicate as closely as possible the original diet of the most primal peoples. The Book of Genesis, for example, indicates that at the beginnings of human history, meat was not eaten at all (Genesis 1:29). Even after man began to kill animals for food, meat was still not a dietary staple, but was usually eaten only on special occasions (Genesis 18:4-8). Even during the days of Jesus, the typical diet consisted of dried fruits and nuts, whole-grain breads, juices and maybe fish. Beef and lamb were reserved for celebrations and holy days (Luke 15:22-23; Mark 14:12). Pork was never eaten, and creamy, sugary, calorie-packed desserts were a regular feature only among the luxuriating super-rich.

As we search for total health, let us recognize that our focus must be on finding and consuming whole, natural, nutrient-dense foods as much as possible. We must strive to find foods that are essentially unaltered after harvesting. In a modern society with so many highly processed foods so readily available, this is not always easy. But if we are to eliminate malnutrition and achieve total health, we must try. We must follow the natural pattern and eat the foods prepared for us by nature under the guiding hand of God, not man.

Even the regular intake of natural foods, however, will not absolutely assure that we are getting adequate nutrition, since even raw, naturally-produced fruits, vegetables and grains can be depleted of essential nutrients due to modern food production methods. So much emphasis has been placed on eye-appeal and efficiency of production that nutrient content has become, at best, a secondary concern. More and more fruits and vegetables are being engineered to improve color, taste, mouth feel, shelf life, harvestability and yield with little attention being given to nutritional content. In many cases, foods that were once considered excellent sources of vitamins are now found to contain only a fraction of their expected vitamin content. For example, oranges have been found with only trace amounts of vitamin C, and carrots have been found with only slight amounts of vitamin A activity.

Even the mineral content of fresh produce has been affected. As crops and grains are harvested year after year, over forty minerals may be stripped from the soil while only a relative few are replaced by conventional fertilizers. Every season the mineral content of much of our farmland is deteriorating. Along with this deterioration comes a corresponding decrease in the mineral content of commercially available fruits and vegetables. Therefore, it is not surprising that studies have demonstrated that the diet of the average American is deficient in a wide range of nutrients, especially minerals.

My point is that even though a diet consisting of properly balanced, fresh, whole foods is the wisest alternative to a diet consisting primarily of highly processed foods, this natural diet may still be nutritionally deficient. Therefore, it may be necessary to consider nutritional supplementation.

## Nutritional Supplements

Although many millions of Americans take nutritional supplements, there are still those who believe that since they do not feel sick, they have no need for supplemental nutrition. The apparent absence of disease, however, is no guarantee of lasting health. Malnutrition does not always manifest itself as an obvious illness; sometimes it takes the form of any of a wide variety of subclinical symptoms such as decreased energy, moodiness, sleeplessness, aggressiveness, increased susceptibility to disease and even obesity. Malnutrition may be the direct cause of virtually any disease, or it may simply be the initiating factor that leads to disease.

Other factors which may contribute to the need for nutritional supplementation are the stresses of work, social stresses, pollution, athletic activity, surgery, and a variety of factors associated with aging. Therefore, for these and many other reasons, I believe there is, generally speaking, a clear need for vitamin/mineral supplementation. But what kind of supplements should we use?

Nutritional supplements are available today in a variety of combinations and dosages, most boasting that they have been scientifically formulated to meet the needs of a specific age group, gender, condition of health, stress or activity. With most manufacturers producing many tablets to choose from, selections can be very confusing, especially for those whose lifestyle suggests the need for more than one type of multivitamin.

Complicating matters further, the nutritional needs of every person is in a continual state of flux. While a megadose of a specific vitamin or mineral may be safe during a time of increased need and decreased consumption, it could become a dangerous excess under other circumstances. That could mean anything from wasted vitamins (and wasted money) to an increased demand on the liver and kidneys. It could even result in harmful toxic effects.

No one actually knows how much of each nutrient is best for any individual at any given time. Recognizing this, the best and safest supplement is one that is closest to the natural state. Just as natural foods are better than foods altered by man, so are natural vitamins and minerals better than the kind that have been extensively processed and packaged by man.

The primary failing of most vitamin/mineral supplements is that they are not prepared for use in a natural form. Instead, they are often only isolated, synthetic vitamins or mineral salts, sometimes mixed with *natural sounding* plants or chemicals. These supplements, regardless of how they may sound, are not natural and are therefore not the best.

It can be argued that synthetic vitamins are chemically identical to their natural counterparts. But in and of itself, the molecular structure of the vitamin or mineral is not what determines the effectiveness of the supplement. Instead, it is the chemical environment of the nutrient that determines its biological activity. Vitamins and minerals are not found isolated in nature; they are always part of complexes. Thus, it is supplements in their natural form and natural balances that are most effective.

Great care should always be exercised when selecting a nutritional supplement. Just as food selections may seem good on the surface yet be nutritionally faulty, so may supplements. The best protection is to choose supplements made by a company which has demonstrated a genuine concern for good nutrition and which supports its products with meaningful literature. When choosing a product, look for a company that is trustworthy and honorable, for this is the best indicator that the product will also be trustworthy and honorable.

## The Need for Clean Water

Although water is not generally considered a nutrient, our bodies are mostly water and water is, therefore, critically important. Yet the water many people drink is filled with impurities and toxic chemicals. It only makes good sense that we should drink only water of the highest quality available. Unfortunately, this leaves out virtually every municipal water system in the country as well as many private wells. The water from most systems contains such contaminates as lead, nitrates, pesticides, industrial waste, microorganisms, inorganic minerals and chlorine. Our bodies were not designed to process these contaminants, and their steady consumption is risky, to say the least.

Total health cannot be achieved and maintained as long as we regularly consume contaminated water. If the quality of the water you drink is in question, consider distilled water. Any additional expense will be well worth it. It is pure water, not contaminated and polluted water, that will contribute the most to our search for total health.

## Don't Forget to Exercise

As with water, physical exercise is generally not considered a part of good nutrition. However, it is so closely connected to the matter of good nutrition and physical health that I must touch on it.

There is no question that the sedentary lifestyle of many Americans is a major contributor to poor health. In days gone by, people walked, and the daily task of life were enough to maintain some measure of physical fitness. Today, for many of us, if we are going to keep ourselves fit, we must work at it.

My purpose is not to go into a long dissertation on how to keep physically fit. Let me just say that many experts say that fitness can be maintained by working out for about twenty to thirty minutes three times a week. That's all it takes for most of us. I am not saying that we all have to be great athletes to enjoy total health, but I am saying that we need to keep our muscles toned and our flab at a minimum.

## Summation

It is simplicity, not complexity, that ought to guide us in our search for total health. If God has, in fact, established the workings of the human frame, then He certainly has established it so that any human being, regardless of intellectual prowess, can understand the basics of staying in good health and free from disease. It almost seems that the more we try to figure it all out, the more confusing the whole issue of health becomes.

I propose that God has established a few basic principles which unfortunately many people are ignoring. I believe that if we would get back to them, we would find that better health awaits us all.

The first principle is that our primary, regular diet should consist predominantly of fresh, whole, natural foods, as free as possible from toxic chemicals and other contaminants. The second is that although ideally we ought to be able to obtain complete nutrition from the foods we eat, we must recognize that in the real world this may not always happen. Therefore, nutritional supplements prepared in a natural environment should be considered in order to be certain that all nutritional requirements are met. The third is that we should drink only the purest water available. And the fourth is that we must get adequate physical exercise, along with plenty of fresh air, sunshine and rest.

The principles I have just enumerated have to do with the nourishment of the physical body—the outward man. So far we have not examined the question as to what constitutes good nutrition for the inward man. This will be our goal in the next chapter.

## Chapter 3

# The Nourishment of the Inward Man

f the health of our physical body is dependent upon being fed wholesome and nutritious food, then what is the health of our spiritual body—our souls—dependent upon? Since our outward man must be nourished properly in order to function properly, I believe the same is true of our inward man. For many, however, their undernourished souls are hindering them from achieving total health and are leaving the door wide open for serious disease.

Webster's Dictionary defines "disease" as: "the lack of ease." It also defines it as: "discomfort, uneasiness, trouble or distress." These terms can apply just as easily to the inward part of man as they can the outward. A gall bladder can be distressed, but so can a mind. A body can be sick, but so can a soul.

The word "soul" refers in a general sense to the inward part of man, including the mind. The Bible often uses the word "soul" in this manner. However, on several occasions the inward man is described as having both soul and spirit, the spirit being the deeper, more subconscious part of the soul.

The Bible describes the functions of these two spiritual organs or systems within the inward part of man. The soul is the self-aware part of man. It is the seat of man's mental and emotional faculties. It is where man's decision-making capabilities lie. Psychologists would consider this roughly equivalent to what they call the conscious mind. The spirit of man is the seat of man's intuition. It is where man becomes aware of the metaphysical world and of God. Psychologists would consider this to be roughly equivalent to what they call the subconscious mind. I believe that the spirit of man, which came directly from God, has an innate super-intelligence which governs the non-conscious inner workings of the physical body, such as the immune system.

According the Bible, these two systems, or spiritual organs, within the inward part of man are extremely difficult to differentiate from one another. Hebrews 4:12 says that it is only the Word of God that can clearly and accurately discern between that which is of the soul and that which is of the spirit. What is clear to me, however, is that what affects the soul affects the spirit and vice versa. Therefore, in this chapter we will not attempt to draw a sharp line between the two, but will simply refer to the inward part of man as the soul or the inward man, understanding that there are many things which significantly impact both parts.

The Bible teaches that what proceeds from the earth—bread—is the food of our outward man. But Jesus never said that man did not live by bread, only that he did not live by bread alone. That which proceeds from God—His Word—is the food for the inward man. It seems to me that it is fair to say that when Jesus spoke of man living by bread, He was using bread to represent food generally, since, like bread, everything we eat originates in the earth. It is also fair, I believe, to say that the Word which proceeds from the mouth of God applies broadly to everything that proceeds from God for our spiritual nourishment. Within this setting I want to discuss the various nutritional needs of our inward man.

## Proper Word Nutrition

"How painful are honest words!" Job said in the midst of his despair (Job 6:25). Words have great power to accomplish both good and ill. This is because words convey thoughts and ideas, and thoughts and ideas are the food of the inward man. The Bible says that "every word of God is flawless" (Proverbs 30:5). Therefore, we can have great assurance that when we feed on the words contained in the Bible, we are feeding our souls on spiritual food which is health-producing and without contamination.

The Prophet Jeremiah said, "When Your words came, I ate them; they were my joy and my heart's delight" (Jeremiah 15:16). The Word of God is nutritionally complete. It is all our souls need in order to thrive and rejoice. Reading, studying, meditating on, and hearing the Word of God preached and taught ought to be a dietary staple as we seek to provide proper spiritual nutrition to our inward man.

A thought or idea can come into our minds, be briefly considered and then depart; or it can come into our minds, be deeply contemplated, and take up residence. It is only those thoughts that take up residence that affect the health of our souls. Therefore, we ought to be careful what we think about and meditate on over a prolonged period of time. We ought to heed Paul's recommendation: "Finally, brothers, whatever is true, whatever is noble, whatever is right, whatever is pure, whatever is lovely, whatever is admirable – if anything is excellent or praiseworthy – think about such things" (Philippians 4:8). This is a fundamental key to good nutrition of the soul.

To suggest that every Christian, or even the most devoted Christian, should read or listen to nothing but the pure, unadulterated Word of God would be to deny the realities of human life. I can't believe even God expects that. What He does expect, however, is that we make the Bible a central part of our lives. But what else constitutes good nutrition for the inward man? Let's examine some possibilities.

Sir John Murray made the observation, "A dose of poison can do its work only once, but a bad book can go on poisoning people's minds for any length of time." What is a "bad book"? Is it one that is poorly written? Or does the quality of a good book have more to do with its substance? I would say the answer is both. I have read books that contained good ideas; yet they were written so poorly that my soul felt more vexed than strengthened. On the other hand, I have read some beautifully written books that left me feeling dirty because the content was dirty. I believe that content is the most important thing we must consider.

It may be all right to eat something from time to time solely because it is enjoyable, but most of the time we ought to eat primarily because it is good for us. If it is enjoyable so much the better. The same holds true for reading. We may occasionally read solely for pleasure, but most of our reading ought to be to increase our knowledge, sharpen our minds, or inspire our hearts. The apostle Paul's position was that just because something was lawful (as opposed to being sinful), did not necessarily mean it constituted a positive spiritual influence (1 Corinthians 10:23). Reading exclusively for entertainment is like trying to be healthy on a diet of chocolate cake.

Tyren Edwards advised, "We should be as careful of the books we read as of the company we keep." This seems to me to be sound advice. Sir Francis Bacon suggested, "Some books are to be tasted; others swallowed;

and some few to be chewed and digested." This also seems like a good guideline to follow.

The printed word is a powerful force for both good and evil. Let us use it for our good. Let us nourish our hearts and minds with reading material that is morally pure, compatible with the basic principles of God's Word, and generally uplifting and inspirational. Let us not allow the adversary to fill our souls with the muck and slime he is using to corrupt the minds of so many in our world today.

## Proper Picture Nutrition

David wrote, "I will set before my eyes no vile thing" (Psalms 101:3). He said this because he understood the great power images have on the state of our souls. Every thing we see affects us either for good or ill. The effect of a fleeting glance may be minimal, but the things we allow to linger before our eyes will truly have a great impact on our spiritual health. Therefore, we must carefully select what we watch on television or in the movies, and we must carefully screen what magazines and other media we expose ourselves to.

Nehru, the first prime minister of India, said: "We seem to pay too much attention to the cinema. It is undoubtedly an excellent medium for many good things, but unfortunately it has not proved to be particularly inspiring." I would say that as of today, this is a severe understatement. And what can be said of the content of television?

Pornography is another branch of the American media. It used to be confined to the sleazy skid-row "adult" bookstores. But today it has infiltrated our local movie theaters, our local convenience stores, and even the daytime television that pours into our own living rooms. Several countries have recognized the extremely detrimental effects pornography has on society and have banned it altogether. I cannot understand why we in America tolerate its profusion into our society. Are we really willing to sit back and watch our civilization be destroyed in the name of protecting the right to free speech?

There are those who think that adults have the capability to see certain things, consciously reject that which is bad, and keep only that which is good. But is that really true? When we feed our body poor food, does it reject the bad and keep only the good? Unfortunately it processes the bad right along with the good—the good building up health and the bad tearing it down. Likewise, our souls keep both good and bad—the good building up our inward man and the bad tearing it down.

The good news in all of this is that we are in charge; we decide what enters in through our eyes over a prolonged period of time and what doesn't. God has given each of us both the ability and responsibility to control what comes into our souls. There are wholesome magazines, movies and television programs available which will nourish our souls. For our health's sake, it is important that each of us as individuals be very selective in what we watch.

## Proper Music Nutrition

Leopold Stokowski once said, "It is not necessary to understand music. Good music, like good food, builds; whereas bad music, like bad food, destroys." Clearly there is a parallel here. If there is bad food which results in poor health, then I believe there is also bad music, which results in poor mental and spiritual health. I'm not certain that I can totally explain how or why this is true, for as Thomas Carlysle said, "The meaning of song goes deep. Who is there that, in logical words, can express the effect music has on us?"

Psychologists have found that music can affect a person whether they want it to or not. For example, it is a fact that fast tempos invariably raise a person's pulse, respiration, and blood pressure while slow music lowers them. Studies have also shown that raucous or inharmonious music has a negative effect on plant growth and on the production of milk cows. Surely we can only wonder at the significance of the effect it may have on humans.

I believe that the best music to listen to is that which expresses something of the majesty, the greatness, the goodness, the peacefulness, the love and the sweetness of the Spirit of Christ. This standard should be applied to both the music itself and the lyrics. Raucous, confused, discordant, harsh or melancholy songs are contrary and adverse to the nature of the gentle Savior. Music that promotes sensuality, violence or rebellion against authority, whether musically or lyrically, should definitely be avoided. Lyrics that promote anti-Christian values or conduct will not be conducive to good spiritual health.

Martin Luther made the statement, "Music is one of the fairest and most glorious gifts of God, to which Satan is a bitter enemy, for it removes from the heart the weight of sorrow, and the fascination of evil thoughts." This may have been the case during his day, but in our modern world, the airwaves are saturated with the devil's music, which actually increases sorrow and fills the minds with evil thoughts. If we are to progress in our search for total health, then we must fill our ears and our hearts only with music that will contribute to a peace-governed, Christ-filled inner man.

## Proper Worship Nutrition

When I speak of worship, I am intending to include everything that is a part of our religious lives—everything that has to do with our relationship with God and our relationships with other people. Concerning our relationship with God, there is good news and there is bad news. First, the bad news: we were all born into this world with a nature inherently bent on rebellion and sin. We inherited this nature from our great-great-great-great (etc.) grandfather, Adam. It is sometimes called "the flesh".

Everyone born since Adam's disobedience has been born without the nature God originally intended for man. Looking at it from the standpoint of spiritual nutrition, our fallen nature hungers for a diet that is harmful rather than wholesome. According to the Bible, all who are without Christ (and many who claim to know Him) feed and sustain themselves on a diet of impure, lustful thoughts, temporal pleasures, materialistic desires (which the Bible calls idolatry), spiritism (that is, encouraging the activity of demons), hatred and fighting, jealousy and anger, constant efforts to satiate every self-centered desire, complaints and criticisms, and such (Galatians 5:19-21). Those who nurture such things in their souls are condemned to living under the dominion of the flesh, that anti-God fallen nature. Left unchanged, the end result is premature death, both naturally and spiritually.

All attempts to correct these symptoms of a diseased soul without dealing with the root appetites will prove vain. But if the appetites change, so will the diet. Let's face it, most of us to some degree eat what we crave. Change the cravings and we change what we eat. But how do we change the cravings? The only way is to change our very nature.

Now, the good news. We don't have to allow the nature we were born with to dominate us. We can place ourselves under the dominion of a new nature. The disobedience of our forefather in the Garden of Eden left us hopelessly incomplete. But the Lord has given hope to every man. He offers everyone a chance to be born again. This second birth, which is provided by Jesus Christ, enables us to become partakers of His own divine nature, which is inherently bent on submission and obedience to God's will (2 Peter 1:4). Since God's will is that we all enjoy total health, as we submit to the new nature that Christ places within us, we will be inspired as never before to move toward our goal of total health.

There is a stark contrast between the two natures I have described: the first produces appetites which lead ultimately to disease and death; the second produces appetites which lead toward maximized health and life. How then does a person become born again and experience the newness that comes with it?

The Bible teaches that all of us have sinned and fallen short of the glory (that is, the perfection) of God (Romans 3:23). The wages of our sin is death (Romans 6:23). Regardless how religious we may try to be or how noble our efforts are to do good works, none of these things can undo the consequences of our sins (Ephesians 2:8-9). They are all nothing more than works of the flesh. The only way we can be saved from our sins is by receiving God's forgiveness and starting all over again. Jesus called this being born again (John 3:3-7).

But Jesus Christ is willing to do more than forgive us and give us another chance; He is also willing to indwell us by His Spirit, imparting to us His own nature and His super-natural power over sin. Paul called this "living a new life" (Romans 6:4).

The Bible teaches that Christ died for our sins to demonstrate His love for us and remove the death penalty that hung over our heads. It teaches that He rose from the dead to demonstrate His power over death and to enable us to partake of His victory. The key to partaking of the risen Christ and His glorious divine nature is submitting to His Lordship.

The apostle James tells us, "Submit yourselves, then, to God ...come near to God and he will come near to you" (James 4:7-8). When God comes near to us, He imparts to us His strength and power to resist temptation. Paul wrote, "So I say, live by the Spirit, and you will not gratify the desires of the sinful nature" (Galatians 5:16). Living by the Spirit is synonymous with submitting to God. It is making Christ the Lord of your life by committing to faithful obedience to His commandments, briefly expressed as loving the Lord with all your heart, mind, soul and strength, and loving your neighbor as yourself (Mark 12:30-31).

These two commandments are the essence of true worship. They speak of our relationships with others and our relationship with God. Both are to be relationships of love. Of all that we do to improve the health of our inward man, let us focus most intently on our worship. If we leave this purely spiritual aspect out of our search for total health, the foundation will be shaky and incomplete. In fact, the achievement of total health will be impossible.

To some the term "born again" may be nothing more than a cliché, but I assure you it is real. To see a person's inherent nature change from one extreme to the other is truly amazing. The prophet Ezekiel described the change this way:

> *I will sprinkle clean water on you, and you will be clean; I will cleanse you from all your impurities and from all your idols. I will give you a new heart and put a new spirit in you; I will remove from you your heart of stone and give you a heart of flesh.* (Ezekiel 36:25-26)

Writing in his classic devotional "My Utmost for His Highest," Oswald Chambers explains the born-again life in a beautiful and profound way. He writes:

> The experience of salvation means that in your actual life things are really altered, you no longer look at things as you used to; your desires are new, old things have lost their power. One of the touchstones of this experience is-has God altered the thing that matters? If you still hanker after the old things, it is absurd to talk about being born again from above, you are juggling with yourself. If you are born again, the Spirit of God makes the alteration manifest in your actual life and reasoning, and when the crisis comes, you are the most amazed person on earth at the wonderful difference there is in you. There is no possibility of imagining that *you* did it. It is this complete and amazing alteration that is the evidence that you are a saved soul.

Let us not confuse this born-again experience with what is called "religion" or "church" or even "cleaning up one's act." I'm talking about a change that occurs deep within a person's heart and produces within him a new perspective and new appetites. Paul said it beautifully when he wrote: "Therefore, if anyone is in Christ, he is a new creation; the old has gone, the new has come!" (2 Corinthians 5:17). Certainly this change must include our deepest, most innate desires. I will be the first to admit that religious observances and mere church attendance cannot accomplish this. Just as the old nature hungered for evil things; the new nature of Christ hungers for righteous things. It longs to be filled with love, joy, peace, patience, kindness and self-control, which are wonderfully nutritious to the soul of man (Galatians 5:22-23).

The old nature isn't equipped to digest such concepts as love and peace and joy. It becomes bothered by them and rejects them. The new nature, however, if we will totally submit ourselves to it, will help us to stay healthy by rejecting such things as envy, anger and hatred.

Perhaps the essence of this new Christ-like nature can be summed up in one word: love. The Bible says, "God is love" (1 John 4:8). Paul wrote a beautiful description of God's love in 1 Corinthians chapter 13. Once this divine love, which only God can give, becomes real in our lives, it causes us to want to fulfill the Lord's commandments to love Him and to love other people. But it also ought to cause us to realize that we are no longer our own. As Paul wrote, "Do you not know that your body is a temple of the Holy Spirit, who is in you, whom you have received from God? You are not your own; you were bought at a price. Therefore honor God with your body" (1 Corinthians 6:19-20).

According to the Bible, we were all sold into sin (Romans 7:14). But because God loved us, He died for us and purchased us with His own blood (Acts 20:28). Therefore, He owns us. We are His personal property. We no longer have the right to feed either our bodies or our souls whatever we want. We are to glorify God in both. We must therefore strive to learn everything that God wants us to know concerning the achievement of total health.

To bring all of this into a more practical light, let me say that I believe that if we are to feed ourselves with proper worship food, it must begin with a daily time of personal devotions and Bible study. We must set aside time every day for just us and the Lord. How can we say we love Him if we are unwilling to spend any time with Him?

Next, I believe we must periodically set aside a time for fasting. This will not only cleanse the soul and increase our desire for spiritual things, but it will also produce a wonderful cleansing of the body. Just a few days of fasting will cause the body to begin a purging process of all accumulated toxic substances, which are there in the first place because of poor nutrition and are major contributors to disease. (There are many good books available on the benefits and procedures of fasting.)

In addition to our individual spiritual exercises, I believe every believer ought to be an active member of a vibrant, Bible-believing congregation. It is not enough to simply study the Bible privately; every one of us also needs to hear the Word of God taught and preached on a regular basis.

We also need a place and structure through which we can learn to live out the things we are learning. Head knowledge of the Scriptures will never be enough; the Lord wants us to also have heart knowledge. This means that we must put the teachings of the Bible into practice. Mental love does a person no good. It is only when love is activated that people are blessed and experience the reality of Jesus Christ.

Furthermore, Jesus taught that it is more blessed to give than to receive. He said this because He understood how greatly the inward man is blessed by giving. Many have testified how the depression they had suffered with for years departed after they got involved in some kind of charitable work. Let us take note that giving selflessly of our time and energy is one of the greatest deterrents to disease available to us.

## Proper Fellowship Nutrition

As I have said, in many ways our relationships with other people are a part of our worship of God. The apostle John wrote, "For anyone who does not love his brother, whom he has seen, cannot love God, whom he has not seen" (1 John 4:20). Therefore, our involvement with God must, of necessity, involve us with other people. But such involvement presents the opportunity for both positive and negative influence.

It ought to be our desire to want to be a positive influence toward all people we come into contact with. But we must consider the reality that those we have contact with will also have an influence on us, either for good or ill. Often the influence may be minimal and may be within what we would consider to be an acceptable range of negative influence. But there will be influence nonetheless.

What we must be particularly concerned with is having prolonged exposure to those who have a particularly negative influence on us. Paul wrote, "Do not be misled; bad company corrupts good character" (1 Corinthians 15:33). He also wrote, "Don't you know that a little yeast works through the whole batch of dough?" (1 Corinthians 5:6). In the first verse Paul was talking about those who promote ideas and doctrines contrary to acceptable Christian beliefs. In the second he was talking about those involved in conspicuous acts of immorality.

In both of these situations, Paul suggested that the power to influence negatively was so strong that the best solution was to cut off contact altogether. There seems to be something about the power of certain negative ideas and practices that is so strong and so insidious that it can infect and disease a whole body of people if it is not removed. This is why Paul instructs, "Expel the wicked man from among you" (1 Corinthians 5:13).

What I am discussing here is not intended to in any way promote division and disunity among believers, or division and distrust between believers and unbelievers. I am only presenting a principle of spiritual health, and it must be received in that context. The fact is, the people we associate with on a regular basis will have a profound effect on our spiritual condition, and potentially on our physical condition. If we associate with people whose faith is strong, whose lives are clean, who walk with the Lord, we will be led along in that direction. But if we associate primarily with people who like to gripe and complain, who gossip about other people, and who run for the medicine chest rather than to Jesus Christ for every little ache or pain, then we will likewise be led in that direction.

Orchids grow best in a hot, wet climate. Cactuses grow best in hot, dry regions. The health and fruitfulness of these plants is determined not only by the nutrition they get, but also by their environment. For a time I had a plaque hanging in my dining room that said, "Bloom where you are planted." This sounds good, but sometimes it's not possible to bloom where you are planted. Perhaps the plaque should read, "Be planted where you can bloom."

The people with whom we associate are our environment. They will either lift us up or drag us down. One group encourages, another discourages. Why not seek out those who will lift us up? Human beings grow and function best in an environment filled with love, peace, and harmony.

Closely related to the influence of other people is the influence we have on ourselves, especially the words we speak. Most of us have a natural tendency to speak critically of other people, to play put-down, to blame others for our own shortcomings and failures, and to generally use our mouths to no good purpose. This is of the flesh. We must begin to take full responsibility for our words, realizing that what we say and often repeat is likely to happen. As a ship is guided by a small rudder and a horse by a tiny bit, so are we guided by our tongues (James 3:3-5). Therefore, let us be careful to speak only positive, health-producing words for the blessing and benefit of our own hearts and minds, as well as the hearts and minds of others.

## Chapter 4

# The Nourishment of Animals and Plants

Gᴏd has given mankind a certain degree of dominion over the animal world, particularly over the world of domestic animals. This dominion carries with it a responsibility to care for our farm animals and pets to the best of our abilities. Proverbs 12:10 says, "A righteous man cares for the needs of his animal." One of the primary ways we as individuals can show proper regard for the lives of whatever animals we may own is by providing them with properly nutritious food. We must recognize that just as proper nutrition is the foundation of human health it is also the foundation of animal health. Therefore, let's look at how well we are meeting our responsibility.

Like human health, animal health is a complex field. Because of this complexity, there is plenty of opportunity for error. However, much error can be avoided by remembering the importance of good nutrition. In determining the proper diet for an animal, the first question should be "What would this animal normally eat in the wild?" Once this question is answered, every effort should then be made to provide that food. Unfortunately, today's approach is all too often "What can we coax our kitty into eating?" or "What's the cheapest (or the most expensive) dog food on the shelf?" There is too little regard for the original, natural diet the animal was created to eat.

We all understand that automobiles run poorly when filled with the wrong fuel. The same can be said of animals. Yes, we can feed them whatever we want to because they are dependent upon us, but wouldn't it be kinder and more beneficial to feed them what they were created to eat? We must play by nature's rules, not our own, if we are to have healthy animals. When we disregard the natural aspects of an animal's diet, we may unknowingly be malnourishing the animal. And once malnutrition occurs, disease will eventually follow.

Just as with humans, animal health is governed by important principles which can guide us in improving the nutrition of our animals. Until knowledge is complete, all we can do is operate as best we can under the umbrella of nutritional principles. For example, some of the principles of nutrition are that ingredients should be whole, that food should contain enzymes and probiotics (pro-life, as opposed to antibiotics, anti-life), that vitamins and minerals should be natural and properly balanced, that food processing should be careful, and that food should be as fresh as possible.

These principles are simple and apply generally to the feeding of all animals, including human beings. I want to apply them specifically, however, to the feeding of pets—especially dogs and cats. The list that follows presents valuable nutritional principles that can be used as criteria for selecting a quality pet food.

## Principle No. 1:
## Whole ingredients are superior to by-products.

Many pet foods contain the by-products of grains and meats. For example, corn is often not whole corn but corn meal, that is, corn without the oils. Rice is frequently rice hulls instead of whole rice. And wheat is often wheat middlings instead of the actual whole wheat. What the label calls "poultry by-products" may be heads and feet and a little viscera instead of actual meat and bones, which is what the animal would normally eat in the wild. The difference between whole ingredients and the fractionated by-products is significant.

## Principle No. 2:
## Food containing probiotics is superior to food without them.

Most of us have been conditioned to believe that all germs are bad and should be destroyed, but this is not true. While some microorganisms do cause harm, others called probiotics are beneficial. In fact, without them our bodies would not function properly. Unfortunately, a variety of stresses can adversely affect the microbial population of the digestive tract. These stresses include sudden food changes, the use of antibiotics and pharmaceuticals, emotional or psychological trauma, the ingestion of chemicals in food or water (many are designed to inhibit bacterial growth such as chlorine, benzoic acid, paraders, sorbates, propionates, sulfites, acetates, and nitrites), exposure to pollution, excessive noise, travel, a change in the environment, continuous exposure to artificial light, excess positive air ions and family upheaval. In essence, just about anything that forces a change in one's natural state of existence can create the stress necessary to disrupt gastrointestinal balances.

Poor human health resulting from microbial imbalances may mean unnecessary suffering and lost work time. For this reason, probiotics are an important dietary supplement for both humans and animals. They can be used to enhance the immune system, inhibit pathogens, decrease disease recovery time and create an overall improvement in health. Probiotics represent a safe and effective alternative to pharmaceutical methods which introduce toxic chemicals foreign to biological experience. The use of probiotics represents a natural preventive and therapeutic approach that is essentially without contradiction.

## Principle No. 3:
## Food containing enzymes is superior to food without them.

Enzymes are the catalysts responsible for a multitude of essential reactions in the body. They have been called the "essence of life", for without enzymes there could be no life. Under normal, natural conditions food contains an abundance of enzymes, but because enzymes are fragile and easily destroyed by excessive heat, cooked and processed foods tend to be severely lacking in them.

The Chinese and Japanese have discovered that enzymes can be produced through the use of healthy microorganisms such as Aspergillus and Bacillus species. These organisms are cultured on various food substrates to produce the enzymes desired. The enzymes are then extracted and dried into a powder. These cultured enzymes are excellent because of their optimum activity in the mildly acidic environment of the upper stomach.

Enzyme supplementation is important for anyone eating cooked or processed foods. Food enzymes result in increased nutrient absorption and more efficient use of nutrients with less demand placed on the enzyme-secreting organs. Good health is not so much a result of what we eat as it is what we actually digest. *An essential feature of all natural foods: they contain enzymes. An essential feature of all processed foods: they do not contain enzymes.* Could this be a key to the mystery of why all degenerative diseases (such as cancer, heart disease or diabetes) increase in societies where processed foods are introduced as a predominant portion of the diet? When raw, natural, enzyme-rich foods cannot be eaten, enzyme supplementation offers an excellent means to restore essential food enzyme features to the modern diet.

## Principle No. 4:
## Natural, God-made vitamins are superior to synthetic, man-made vitamins.

There are some who insist that a vitamin is a vitamin, regardless of its origin. But research has proven that natural vitamins are absorbed five times better and are retained six times better than synthetics. Also, in contrast to a purified synthetic chemical, natural source vitamins carry with them associated biochemicals and minerals as cofactors, as well as unknowns that are believed to enhance and broaden the action of vitamins. It should be remembered that in nature vitamins are not found in isolated forms; they are balanced with other vitamins and nutrients in complex interrelationships. Therefore, it seems wise to put our trust in God and seek to ingest vitamins packaged as closely as possible to the way He originally planned.

## Principle No. 5:
## Organic minerals are superior to inorganic minerals.

Recent evidence has suggested that minerals play a far greater role in metabolism than previously thought. Research has also shown that minerals in their original, organic forms are better absorbed and more bioavailable then minerals in inorganic forms. Furthermore, studies have indicated that the organics are more effectively stored within the body for future needs than the same amounts of minerals in the inorganic form. Thus, as with vitamins, minerals in their natural, organic complexes do the most to enhance our health.

## Principle No. 6:
## Natural preservation is superior to chemical preservation.

Foods can be preserved with chemical preservatives such as BHA and BHT, but recent research is showing these antioxidants to be potentially harmful. It is true that when no preservatives are added, problems with rancidity and toxicity may arise, especially when food containing valuable oils and fats spoils and breaks down. Therefore, packaged foods should definitely be preserved, but preferably not with synthetic preservatives. Natural herbal extracts and vitamin epimeres are a safe and effective means of food preservation and stabilization.

## Principle No.7:
## Gentle, low heat processing is superior to harsh high-heat processing.

The nutrient value of food can be virtually destroyed by such processing procedures as high heat, mechanical forces, solvent extraction, distillation, oxidation and hydrogenation. Processing should therefore be done carefully and with concern for nutrient preservation. Proper processing enables food to remain as close as possible to its natural state, making it of greater value to the animal or person eating it.

When selecting a pet food, the principles of wholeness, probiotics, enzymes, natural vitamins, organic minerals, natural preservatives and careful processing should be considered and used as guide for choosing the right food. To help, the following questions might be asked: Is this food made with whole ingredients or by-products? Does it contain probiotics? Are the enzymes dead or alive? Are the vitamins natural or synthetic? Are the minerals organic or inorganic? Are the preservatives chemical or natural? Was the processing gentle or harsh and is the food fresh? Additionally, it is important to remember that pets (dogs and cats) are carnivores, and meat is part of their natural diet. Keep in mind also that animals, like humans, need clean and pure water. These principles can serve as practical guides for choosing the best foods and thereby enhancing your pet's health.

In conclusion, let us remember that knowledge is in a constant state of development. Until we know everything necessary to formulate a perfect food, we should use nature as our guide and put our trust in God's ways. He, after all, has been feeding animals for thousands of years and surely knows more about nutrition than we do. Essentially it comes down to making a choice between the ways God has established in nature and the ways man has created through his own intelligence. Would you rather stake the health and well-being of your animals and your family on God, or on man?

## Plant Health

It has been said that agriculture is the backbone of civilization. This is a strong statement, yet worthy of consideration, for without agriculture there would be no food, and without food there would be no civilization. And just as it is possible to feed human beings poorly and produce unhealthy people, so it is possible to feed plants poorly and produce unhealthy plants. Thus the question arises: are we feeding our plants as we should? If plants are fed less than the best, they may grow up looking good, but they may not be as healthy as they should be. For example, they may not contain the nutrients necessary to fulfill their purpose of nourishing the animals and the people who consume them. In other words, if plants are fed poorly, they will be weak and sickly, which will ultimately result in weak, sickly animals and people. The importance of plant health and proper plant nourishment cannot be overemphasized.

According to the Bible, the physical substance of plants, animals and people all have the same origin: the earth (see Genesis 2:7, 9, 19). This explains why the same essential elements that are found in plants, animals and people are also found in earth. Furthermore, plants, animals and people can all suffer some of the same deficiencies. For example, each can suffer a calcium deficiency, each can suffer an iron deficiency, and each can even suffer a boron deficiency. The similarities and relationships between our health and the health of plants and animals are far greater than most people realize. If plants are to be healthy they must be fed properly, like animals and people. Otherwise, malnutrition will develop and disease will result.

Animals and people are healthiest when fed natural, God-made foods. The same is true of plants. It is possible to produce crops using man-made fertilizers, but crops nourished with natural fertilizers such as manure and compost will be healthier and more productive.

In conclusion, just as nutrition is the foundation of human and animal health, it is also the foundation of plant health. If it makes a difference what foods we feed ourselves and our animals, then it also makes a difference what foods we feed our plants. To reiterate, agriculture is the backbone of civilization. Therefore, we must strive as a society to produce the most healthy, nutrient-rich plants we can.

## Chapter 5

# The Mission

Several years ago, I heard a teacher speak on the subject, "How to Determine Your Mission in Life." At the close of his presentation he asked that all who wanted to know God's will for their lives come forward so he could pray for them. It surprised me to see how many people went forward, even those later in life. Evidently everyone, regardless of age, needed guidance and direction in finding their mission in life.

After his prayer the teacher encouraged everyone to devote the days that followed to asking God to reveal to them what their life's mission was all about. We were then to write it down in a minimal number of words. I did as instructed and this is what I wrote:

"My mission in life is to have a positive influence on world health. This influence is to be in the field of nutrition and is to include the effects of nutrition on plants, animals, and people."

I was stunned. What a task! Who was I to think that I could accomplish such a lofty goal? World health? Plants, animals, people? After all, I was only a veterinarian in a small town in rural south Georgia. As time passed, however, I gave considerable thought to this mission and finally decided that I had not dreamed this up myself; I only wrote what came from my heart. I therefore determined to believe that the words and the mission were of God.

As I reread and pondered this mission, I began to notice the word "influence." The mission was "to have a positive *influence* on world health." Before long this mission began to shift in my heart from the utterly impossible to the very possible. After all, the mission was not to correct everything that was wrong in the field of health all by myself. It was simply to influence it to some degree in a positive direction, presumably with the help of the Lord. So my mind began to churn as I started to consider how this might actually come about. I was still aware, however, that I was only a veterinarian in a small town in southern Georgia.

Later on the idea for this book came along. I began to see that with a book I could share information and possibly have the influence I was called to have. Furthermore, I could appeal to people around the world to support the call for better health. If each person touched by this book would commit to improving his or her own health and then help a few other people do the same, what a difference one veterinarian writing one book could make!

The idea of people all over the world becoming stronger and more complete in their bodies, minds and spirits is a wonderful dream and one that is certainly worth working toward. It may be that some would be unable to influence the health of animals or plants or even other people, but surely everyone could do something to improve their own health, and that, after all, is the place to start.

## The Need for Wholeness

Over the years I have become immensely concerned about the lack of proper nutrition and how it relates to our failure as a society to achieve total health. I have also become concerned about the general failure to appreciate the importance of the relationship between the parts and the whole. There are those who scoff at my concerns and consider my positions to be unorthodox; but I believe that what I am presenting in this book is actually more reasonable than most traditional approaches to dealing with health.

Regardless of what I believe or what others may think about what I believe, it is undeniably the case that the trend today is towards more and more specialization with more and more attention being given to the parts and less and less attention being given to the whole. As I have said before, the danger in this approach is that it tends to focus on the intricacies of the parts while neglecting their relationship to other parts and to the whole.

There is nothing intrinsically wrong with specialization, but the functioning of the individual parts is also improved when they are considered in light of the whole. It is often the correctness of the interrelationships between the parts that makes the difference.

In matters of both physical and spiritual health, these relationships grow and become strong when they are receiving proper nutrition. The better the quality and completeness of the nutrition, the better and stronger the relationships. Nutrition is therefore unquestionably the foundation of total health.

God created the world in which we live to function as an organized, harmonious whole. Without this organization—this balance between the constituent parts—it would be only a matter of time before everything would crumble into utter chaos. Likewise, our total health depends upon balance and harmony. It is not enough to eat right, exercise, and get plenty of fresh air and sunshine. If we are to have genuine and lasting health, there must be a harmonious relationship between the physical, the mental, and the spiritual domains.

Imagine a person perched on a three-legged stool, with one leg representing the physical, one the mental, and one the spiritual. Together they provide us with balanced support for a healthy and productive life. Our whole reason for being is to grow to maturity and successfully accomplish the course God has set before us. No one is here by accident. God gave each of us an allotment of time by explicit design. Each of us has a God-ordained reason and purpose for living. We can fail to fulfill it; or we can fulfill it entirely. The latter is God's will. Yet how many will fall short because they have cut short one or more of the legs on their stool?

It is not God's will that any of us simply muddle through life. God has ordained that we be whole, that we be effective, that we achieve and overcome. For this we need total health, which will depend largely upon the proper and balanced nourishment of both our outward and our inward man. Unless there is this balance, wholeness and effectiveness will suffer. Each leg of the stool must be straight and strong. Each must be the same length. Weakness or incompleteness in any of the three legs will result in shakiness and instability. It is not enough to have one or two healthy legs: all three must be healthy. Any combination of long and short, weak and strong, balanced and unbalanced, will lead sooner or later to deterioration and premature collapse.

It is not uncommon to find people who eat right, exercise, and in general take good care of their body. Neither is it uncommon to find people who appreciate their mind, being careful to nourish it with good and edifying thoughts. Furthermore, there are those saints of God who nourish their spirits by regularly reading God's Word, spending time in church and in fellowship with other believers. This is all well and good, but my message is this: unless we give diligent attention to all three legs of our symbolic stool, we will be less-than-our-best, frequently wobbling and at some point toppling over.

Most people admire a healthy body, respect a sharp mind, and are sobered in the presence of a truly godly person. But to see balance in all three areas with its resultant total health is indeed rare. If I could be bold and suggest a goal for all of us, it would be that we have the body of an athlete, the mind of a scholar, the spirit of a disciple, and that all three be in perfect balance. This is neither an impossible nor unrealistic goal. The closer we get to our goal, the closer we are to total health.

The apostle John wrote, "Dear friend, I pray that you may enjoy good health and that all may go well with you, even as your soul is getting along well" (3 John 2). Here we see clearly the relationship between the outward man and the inward man. Our physical health and fitness is intimately tied to our soul's health and fitness, both mentally and spiritually.

Solomon wrote, "My son, pay attention to what I say; listen closely to my words. Do not let them out of your sight, keep them within your heart; for they are life to those who find them, and health to a man's whole body" (Proverbs 4:20-22). To divorce the physical from the spiritual, the spiritual from the mental, the mental from the physical, is foolish indeed. We must see to it that we receive proper nutrition in each area of our lives if we are ever to complete our search for total health.

For most, foundations are not very exciting. Because they are unseen, they tend to be taken for granted or even ignored. Most people get more excited about decorating their house than they do about laying the foundation. But unless the foundation is laid, there is no house. And unless the foundation is solid and stable, the house and the decorations will all one day collapse. Similarly, treating a disease attracts more attention than preventing it. To many, prevention seems dull and boring. Nevertheless, it is far and away better than treatment. Unfortunately, this is a lesson many are only learning through much pain and suffering.

Furthermore, just as good nutrition is the foundation of prevention, it is also the best foundation for treatment. To seek a restoration to health without making the very foundation a top priority is pure vanity, and at best it is only a temporary solution. Yet I am continually amazed at how many people prefer submitting to the blade of the surgeon rather than changing their eating habits or making a deeper commitment to the Lord.

Some may question what I have said about how the health of the inward man affects physical health and fitness. Some may even deny that man has a spirit, arguing that man has only a mind. But I submit that the failure to properly nourish the innermost part of the inward man, the spirit, is the greatest failing today of society in general concerning health.

Some may question my assertion that only that which proceeds from God (specifically the God of the Bible) constitutes proper nutrition for the human spirit. After all, there are many other religions and philosophies in the world, and who can say which is really best? Allow me to respond by saying that Christianity is not merely one of the world's many religions. In fact, true Christianity is not a religion at all; it is a relationship—not just between people, but between individuals and Jesus Christ. That relationship, strengthened by the indwelling Spirit of God, creates a hunger that can be satisfied only by God's word. Other diets may sound good and look good, but they do not truly nourish. And without full nourishment there is malnutrition, which will ultimately lead to disease, destruction, and death. God's Word, on the other hand, leads to true nourishment, full strength and abundant life.

The Bible talks often of the nourishing effects of the Scripture. It instructs us to "Like newborn babies, crave pure spiritual milk, so that by it you may grow up in your salvation" (1 Peter 2:2). If our inward man is to grow to maturity, we must not accept substitutes; we must feed ourselves the things which proceed from God.

The health of the spirit is important, not only because it effects our spiritual well-being (including our eternal life), but also because it effects the other aspects of health as well. Depression, for example, is evidence of a diseased spirit. Moreover, a depressed person usually begins to think wrong. He may even begin to think about suicide, a mental process hardly conducive to good health. Often a depressed person will not eat right or get adequate exercise, thus fueling a decline in physical health. You see, it all works together. To treat depression only on the level of the physical by administering drugs is to shut the sufferer up in prison, barring him from ever proceeding any farther along the pathway that leads to total health.

The message is clear: Total health means much more than just a healthy body; it means a healthy soul as well. And a healthy soul means more than just a healthy mind; it also means a healthy spirit. Our thinking must be right, but our heart must be right as well. This healthy spirit can only be initiated through the experience of the New Birth. Then, as the inward man is nourished by the Word and Spirit of God, and the outward man is nourished by wholesome foods and a wholesome lifestyle, we should expect to begin approaching total health.

## The Challenge

Knowledge is not enough. It is important; it is a prerequisite; it is a good place to start; but knowledge alone is not enough. Along with knowledge there must be action. If we are to achieve total health, we must take what we have learned and put it into action. Knowing and not doing will get us nowhere. The challenge, therefore, is to learn and then apply what we have learned.

To act upon what we have learned means that change must take place. Unfortunately, many people instinctively resist change. For some reason many of us see change as synonymous with loss and therefore fight against it. But is change really loss? It could be, I suppose, but many times change results in a plus. The key is deciding if a thing is good or not, and if it is, working to make use of its goodness. We must realize that the application of goodness will not always be easy, because worthwhile things are seldom easy. I suggest we begin right now cultivating an attitude that will embrace rather than resist the changes we need to make.

To apply the principles of health presented in this book will require effort—determined effort. Old habits must be broken and replaced by new and better ones, and this will not always be fun or easy. It will require commitment; it will require setting goals; it will require persistence; and it will require time to reprogram and establish a better system. Nevertheless, it can be done, and the reward is better health.

There will be distractions, especially from your peers. They will apply pressure and most likely accuse you of becoming fanatical. But which is more important, disdainful comments or better health? Besides, to those who are malnourished and unhealthy, the straight and narrow ways always appear to be fanatical. But the rewards of total health are lasting beyond measure. I encourage you to accept the challenge and give your very best towards becoming a better balanced and better nourished person.

Once our personal health begins to improve and we find that we are heading toward our goal—the body of an athlete, the mind of a scholar and the spirit of a disciple—we must then begin to reach out and help others learn what we have learned. The possibility of achieving total health is good news, and good news should be told. We first must find and apply the principles for ourselves, but then we must teach them to others!

The plan is simple: we learn and teach others, who learn and teach others, who learn and teach others. On and on the progression goes, until the search for total health becomes a widespread phenomenon, sweeping across every corner of society. Remember that ultimately it is *action* that makes the difference. We must teach and encourage others to *act* on what has been taught. Our own successes will serve to demonstrate the possibility of progress. The alternative is to continue on the downhill path and watch as our world, our plants, our animals, and our own lives slowly but surely come apart and sink into oblivion.

I had a friend who once told me an encouraging story of a time when he was younger and had an idea to establish a home for needy people. He pondered and planned, and when the idea had reached maturity in his own heart, he presented it to the proper committee for consideration. Well, as sometimes happens with committees, they were not nearly excited about his plan as he was, and they voted against it. To them it was just another good idea, and they had heard many "good ideas." To my friend, however, It was far more than just another good idea, for by then it had become a dream, a vision and a calling to him. He had no intention of giving it up, especially since it could help so many people.

So my friend persisted, and the committee refused. And when he persisted again, the committee refused again. Then one day he stood before them with unusual determination and dramatically declared, "I will continue to pursue the establishment of this home in full confidence that it will be established, for right is right since God is God, and right the day shall win. To doubt would be disloyalty, to falter would be sin."

The committee began to listen. Perhaps for the very first time they realized that my friend was serious and deeply committed to his vision. His proposal was reconsidered and another vote taken. This time the plan was approved and the home was established.

Today, over sixty years later, that home stands as a standard by which other homes are measured. Its influence touches directly or indirectly the lives of thousands of people every day. Astonishing things can happen when people are willing to stand for what is right.

My appeal for a renewed and enthusiastic search for total health through improved nutrition is a cause that is right. By taking a stand together for what is right, we can improve the nutrition and health of our plants, our animals, and ourselves and by doing so we can then touch and change the lives of others all across our nation and our world. I therefore appeal to all who read this book to take the knowledge and understanding you have acquired and with it pursue the establishment of better health, with full confidence that it can and must be established.

> For right is right
> Since God is God,
> And right the day shall win.
> To doubt would be disloyalty,
> To falter would be sin.

I encourage us all to stand firm for the truth and to run with patience and persistence the race that is set before us.

**Part Two**

---

# A Plan for Better Health

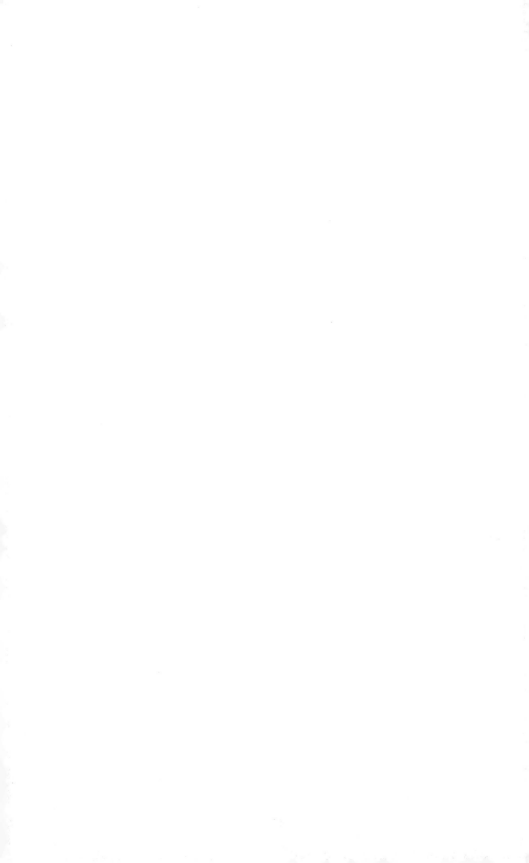

# Introduction

If the question was asked, "Who wants to be healthy?" certainly everyone would say, "I do." If the question was asked, "What is your plan for being healthy?" most would hesitate, think for a moment, and say something like, "Well, I try to take care of myself and if I get sick I go to the doctor." This is the plan followed by nearly everyone, but how is it working? With things like heart disease, cancer and obesity out of control in our country, maybe we should rethink our present plan because it is simply not working!

It has been said that if you keep on doing what you've been doing, you'll keep on getting what you've been getting. Surely we don't want what we've been getting, so we must change. We need a new plan.

## History

I graduated from Auburn University as a veterinarian in 1963 and went out into the world to "make a difference." I was going to use my knowledge and skills to help animals, as I had been trained to do. But I soon saw I could not help as much as I had hoped. It seemed that all too often in the battle against disease, disease won. Why couldn't I win more often? It seemed like something, something basic and essential, was missing, but what?

In the spring of 1977, I learned of a vitamin-mineral-enzyme product for cattle that for some reason I decided to investigate. The company was gracious enough to send me several hundred pounds of the nutritional supplement and I soon saw amazing results! In only days after adding the product to the rations of cows and calves, I observed noticeable improvements. Diarrhea stopped, eyes became brighter, hair coats improved and the animals went from sickness to health right before my eyes! At first I thought it was my imagination but after many trials on many farms over many months I was convinced that the missing ingredient in the formula for health was nutrition!

Living in a rural area and being a veterinarian who worked with both large and small animals, I began to test this cattle product on other species. First horses, then hogs, then dogs, then cats, sheep, goats, chickens, even elephants, and all showed improvements when the product was added to their diet. No longer did I think my findings were in my mind. They were real!

This all led to research projects, published papers, presentations, new products, eventually a book, and a question: "If so many different species of animals could be helped by simply improving their nutrition, what about people? Could people also be helped by improving their nutrition?"

Over the years I continued to ponder my findings and grow in my conviction that proper nutrition was not only critically important, but lacking in most species. My thinking further expanded to realize that people are more than a body. We have a mind and a spirit as well! Furthermore, if a person is to be healthy, totally healthy, each of the 3 parts must be properly nourished.

In the summer of 2001 I received a special invitation: I was invited to Europe (Austria) to speak as a participant in the World Congress for Humanity in Medicine, and I was to speak about my book! I felt honored by this invitation, but I was also apprehensive because my book was as much about feeding the spirit (and the mind) as it was about feeding the body. How could I "preach" to these people from different countries and cultures who had different beliefs and likely different religions without offending them? How could I convey my message of total health in a clear, easy-to-understand way that would help them see health in a different and broader way?

As I thought about this, it came to me that I should tell them a story: a parable.

A parable has been defined as a simple story with a deep meaning. A parable can be so simple that almost anyone can understand it and at the same time it can be so deep and thoughtful that almost no one can understand it, at least not fully. Jesus' parable of the prodigal son (Luke, Chapter 15) is an example of this and a masterpiece that has been called the greatest short story ever written. Thus the power of a parable should not be underestimated.

It is the judgment of most thinking men that man is a trinity: we are body, mind and spirit! This is not a new thought because for thousands of years, from ancient times to modern times, men have written and spoken of us as being body, mind and spirit. But what do we do with this information? Is it merely for philosophical discussion or is it for practical purposes? I suggest it is for practical purposes because if nutrition is the foundation of our physical health, shouldn't it also be the foundation of our mental and spiritual health? If we must feed *one* part, shouldn't we also have to feed *all* parts? Furthermore, all parts are intertwined so that the feeding, or the lack of feeding, of one part affects all parts.

Now, the parable:

# The Parable of the 3-Legged Stool

**R**emembering that man is a trinity and using our imagination, when a child is born they are, figuratively speaking, like a stool:

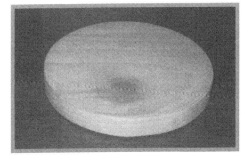

Granted, this does not look like a stool, but as the mother nourishes and cares for the child, the physical leg of the stool begins to grow...

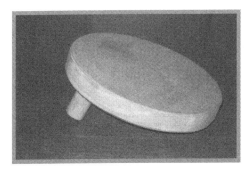

Later there is evidence of mental growth as the child further responds to care and attention. Thus the mental leg is growing...

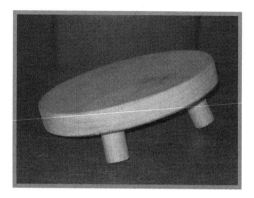

More realistically, the physical leg grows much, with the mind and spirit growing less noticeably.

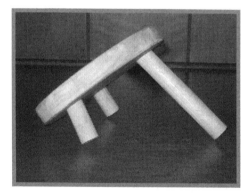

Teenagers are often like this. They are strong in their body, but often lack focus, and have little interest in spiritual matters.

It has been said that life beings at 40 and perhaps it does because as a person approaches 40 they often begin to sense something is missing. On the outside everything looks good. They are married, have 2 children, 2 cars, 2 jobs and a nice house. Still, on the *inside*, something is missing.

As they seek to fill this emptiness they decide to get in better physical shape. They begin to watch their calories, carbs and cholesterol, even exercise some. And before long, they feel better. Their physical leg is growing...

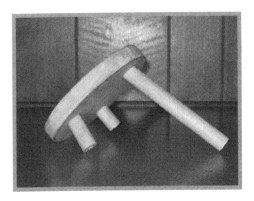

Now, as the "new person" begins to emerge, they decide to go further and get more education. They go back to school, hoping that perhaps more education would fill the unexplained and nagging emptiness. Nevertheless, as the mind is fed, it grows:

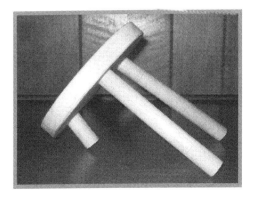

Feeling better about themselves, the person begins to attend church regularly. They had already been going on special occasions but now they feel because of their desire to do better they should attend on a regular basis. Thus, they begin to nourish their spirit and their spiritual leg begins to grow...

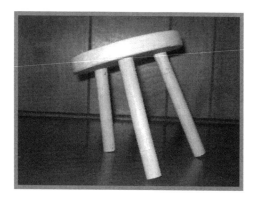

The Bible says we should examine ourselves and upon examination progress is evident. Balance is lacking, but progress is being made and this, of course, is a good thing.

––––––––––––––––

Years ago I was talking with a friend who told me something I had never heard before and have never heard since. This is what he said:

> *"Some men die by hand grenades,*
> *Some go down in flames,*
> *But most men die bit by bit, playing little games."*

One day, hopefully, something happens that causes a person to decide: "No more games." From now on they are serious about their health. From now on they are serious about caring for and nourishing all 3 legs of their "stool." They can't be concerned about what others may think; their concern is to be healthy, as healthy as possible.

## First, feeding the body

2,500 years ago Hippocrates, the Father of Medicine, said "Nutrition is the foundation of health." If this is true, and it is, what should we feed ourselves? What should we feed our bodies? There are so many questions to answer:

- Should I drink soft drinks? Many diet drinks contain aspartame, a harmful excitotoxin.

- Should I become a vegetarian? There are many books on this subject and study is encouraged.

- What about meat? According to the Bible, meat is either clean or unclean. Clean meat can be eaten; unclean meat should not be eaten. (See Leviticus, Chapter 11)

- Should I fast? Fasting is a form of cleansing and detoxification and study on this subject is encouraged.

- Is organic food better? *Warning:* Food additives such as artificial sweeteners, MSG, chemical preservatives and sodium nitrite are, to say the least, not good for humans or animals.

- Are genetically modified foods safe? *Note:* These foods are illegal in many countries of the world.

- Should I get a juicer and make my own fresh fruit and vegetable juice?

- Are microwave ovens safe? They, by the way, have been called "the Kiss of Death" and are prohibited in certain countries of the world.

- Are cell phones safe?

- Are vaccines safe? Are they effective?

- Are the essential oils of the Bible beneficial? These oils have been used for health and healing for thousands of years, and are worth consideration. *Note:* The skin is an absorbing organ, therefore, whatever is put *on* the skin (soaps, shampoos, deodorants, cosmetics...) is absorbed *through* the skin and thus throughout the body! For this reason natural products are best.

- Are nutritional supplements needed?
- What are the fundamentals that I should really focus on?
  - *Natural food.* Fresh fruits and vegetables, as raw as possible. Nuts.
  - *Pure water.* Since our bodies are mostly water we should drink plenty of water, not water with chemicals and contaminants, but plenty of *pure* water.
  - *Laughter.* "A cheerful heart is good medicine." (Proverbs 17:22)
  - *Rest.*
  - *Exercise, fresh air and sunshine.*

This list is incomplete. It is intended only as a beginning; a start that causes a person to think and carefully consider what they are feeding their body.

To learn more about the feeding of the body, you are encouraged to visit www.wysong.net and study the writings and recordings of Dr. R. L. Wysong (If ordering Wysong products, human or animal, call 1-800-748-0188 or order online. Mention code "CC104" for free shipping on your first order).

Now, because of diligence and an attitude of "no more games," our physical leg has become strong and healthy.

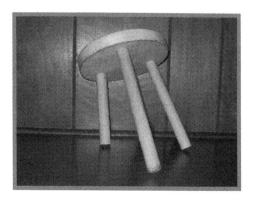

## Second, feeding the mind

Once more the list could be long, but here is a beginning:

- Positive thoughts, realizing that a man becomes what he thinks about.

- Closely related to our thoughts are our own words. Don't speak negative words to yourself or others; speak positive and encouraging words.

- Associate with wise and positive people and benefit from their wisdom and influence.

- Carefully consider what kind of books we read, and the movies and TV programs that we watch.

- Fill your life with positive and stimulating things to expand the mind and soul, such as:

  - *Travel.* To explore other countries and cultures can feed, broaden and strengthen our minds.

  - *Music.* An 18th century Scottish philosopher once said: "You write the laws of your country and I'll write the music. And with the music I will control your country." The kind of music we listen to will greatly influence us, nourishing our minds for better or for worse. I encourage us all to make it for the better.

  - *Attitude.* An attitude that is positive and thankful is essential.

  - *Encouragement.* Words of encouragement can do wonders for a person.

  - *Hope.* Hope and optimism are wonderful and nourishing to the mind.

As before, we examine ourselves and see that progress is being made:

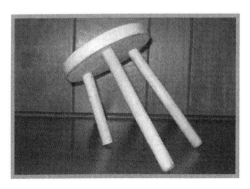

To learn more about the care and feeding of the mind visit www.ziglar.com and study the writings and recordings of Zig Ziglar.

## Third, feeding the spirit

To begin, it should be said that we—all of us—are born with a "heart problem." Because of Adam and Eve and the original sin, we are born with a hard, stony heart that cares mostly for self and little for others. But, if we are to be healthy, this diseased heart must be removed and replaced with a new one! In other words, mankind needs a heart transplant. Individually and collectively we all need new spiritual hearts.

At the meeting in Austria in 2001 the special guest and keynote speaker for the Congress was Dr. Christiaan Barnard, the South African heart surgeon who on Dec. 3, 1967 performed the world's first heart transplant. Meeting Dr. Barnard and hearing him speak helped me see that if man sometimes needs a new physical heart, he might also need a new spiritual heart. How then do we get a new spiritual heart?

Jesus gives us a new spiritual heart. When a person becomes a Christian and accepts Jesus as their Lord and Savior there is a change of heart. The old, diseased heart is replaced with a new one, a new one that is soft and tender. And with a new heart comes a new appetite—an appetite for things like love, joy, peace, patience, kindness, gentleness and hunger for God's word, the Bible. The prophet Jeremiah said "when Your words came I ate them; they were my joy and my heart's delight" (Jeremiah 15:16). And we are told by the apostle Peter "like newborn babies, crave pure spiritual milk, so that by it you may grow up in your salvation" (1 Peter 2:2).

So with a new heart and a hunger for God's Word, our Spirit begins to grow:

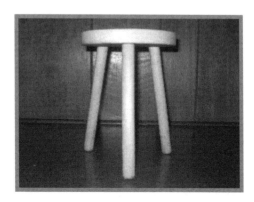

Finally, we have 3 strong legs and a stool that is balanced.

To learn more about the care and feeding of the spirit, you are encouraged to read and study the teachings of the Holy Bible.

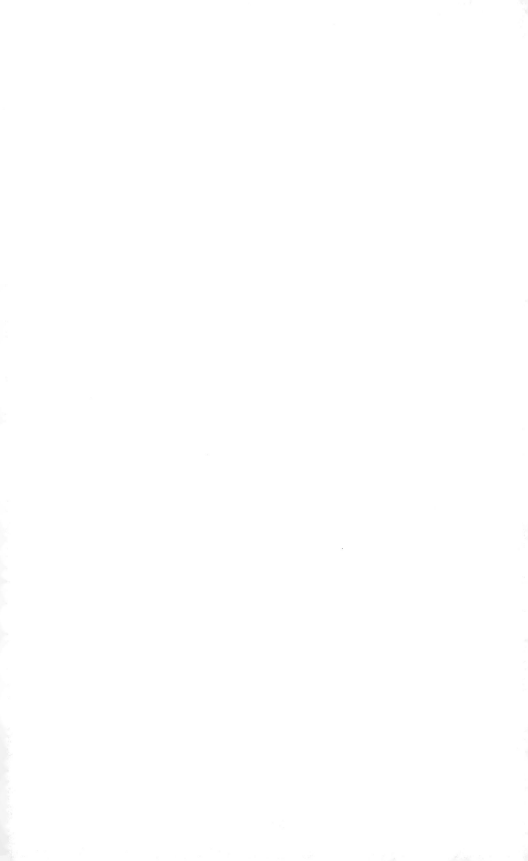

# The Plan

N ow to summarize the plan, the plan that leads to better health. Because we are a trinity, and because nutrition is the foundation of health, the plan that leads to better health is simply this:

*To feed the body God's food: food that is
whole, fresh and unadulterated.*

*To feed the mind godly thoughts: thoughts
that are pure, lovely and admirable.*

*And to feed the spirit God's Word: the Bible.*

# Epilogue

I once read that there are 4 laws of learning: explanation, demonstration, correction and repetition. The parable of the 3-legged stool includes all 4 of these laws.

When the parable is read or heard, the plan is *explained*: Law #1. Pictures, or the stool itself, *demonstrate* the message: Law #2. Next, there is *correction*: Law #3. Correction occurs as poor habits and poor foods are replaced by good habits and good foods. As more and more is learned, more and more corrections can and should be made. Additionally, and this is important, correction is a constant and never-ending task! Lastly is *repetition*: Law #4. Once the plan is understood (through explanation and demonstration) and corrections have been made, the message must be repeated over and over, again and again until it is ingrained in both the conscious and subconscious mind.

# Post Script

For those who have a desire to help, I offer the following thoughts:

The principle of exponential growth is a powerful principle. To understand this principle, and its power, take a penny and double it every day for 1 month. At day one you have 1 cent , at day 2 you have 2 cents, at day three, 4 cents… In the beginning this is near nothing, but as exponential growth continues these few cents grow in 31 days to over $10 million dollars!

When this message is shared with others, who share it with others, who share it with others… in no time at all an enormous number of lives can be touched. And it can all start with just one person: one person who cares about people and spreading the message of better health.

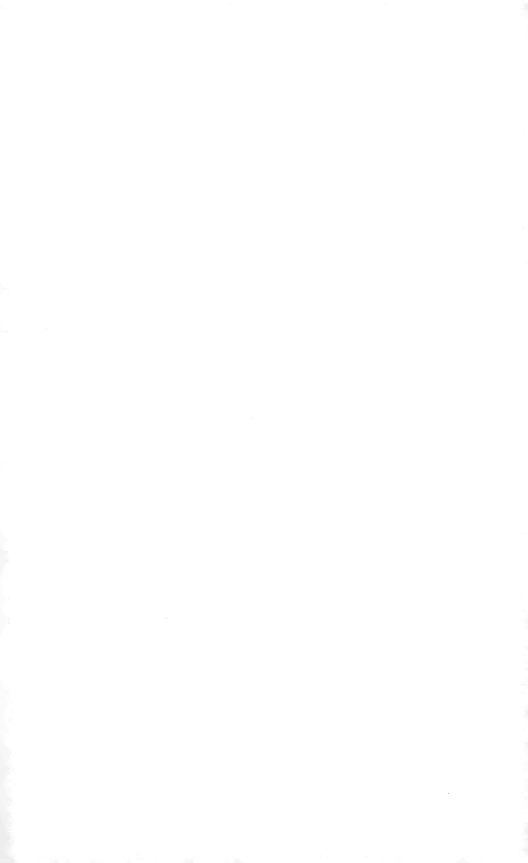

Made in the USA
Columbia, SC
27 April 2022